Is Palliative Care Right For YOU?

By Kevin Haselhorst, MD
Emergency physician and expert on advance care planning

ISBN: 978-0-9915714-2-0

Who knew health care could be so complicated?

- Patients with dementia, heart disease or cancer

- Family caregivers receiving mixed messages about viable treatments

- Healthcare professionals reluctant to discuss death and dying

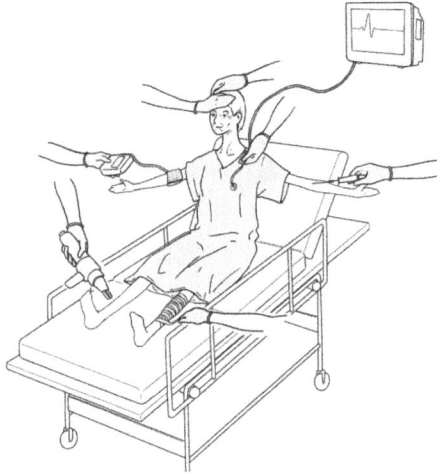

*Living and Dying
should not be as stressful
as the healthcare industry makes it!*

Learn how to make medical decisions less complicated by understanding palliative care. It best serves chronically-ill patients who choose to stay at home. Physicians often recommend these patients call 911 and be hospitalized.

This booklet gives patients permission to break from traditional medical care and focus on their well-being. It introduces "Palliative Care 2.0," which outlines patient goals and personal values.

Contents

Struggling with an incurable illness, you deserve to be treated with compassion. You deserve palliative care.

Palliative care helps patients with serious and chronic illnesses, and their caregivers, control their pain and suffering. It mainly serves retirees who are health-conscious and not beholden to physicians. Palliative care emphasizes listening to patient instead of conducting unnecessary tests and prompts advance care planning prior to emergency room visits. It serves as the bridge between advance and end-of-life care.

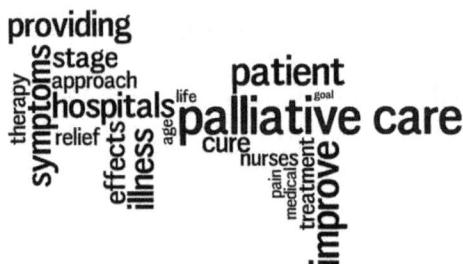

providing stage approach patient therapy symptoms hospitals life palliative care relief effects illness age cure nurses pain medical treatment improve goal

The healthcare system, like a hammock, is nearly impossible to get out of as you become older and weaker. Even at the point when you've had enough, doctors and hospital staff are still afraid to give you permission to die. They perform CPR on everyone who doesn't have an advance directive or a do-not-resuscitate (DNR) order.

Family members want to act in your best interest, but they are hesitant and don't always know your wishes.

What options do you have? **A palliative nurse to the rescue!**

A palliative nurse is highly skilled at listening. This "angel of mercy" opens the door to natural, homeopathic ways of treating illness. Traditional medical care often obliges the chronically-ill to consider options for artificial life support and to be admitted to the hospital. Those who receive palliative care understand their underlying medical condition will not get better and might gladly accept a permission slip from their physicians to remain at home. With a palliative nurse's support, you have a say in how your remaining time and money are spent.

The Two Sides to Your Thinking
Medical Care vs. Palliative Care

Left Brain Medical Care	**Right Brain Medical Care**
Physical Health	Spiritual Well-Being
Healthcare Professionals	Family Caregivers
Medical Intellect	Parental Instincts
Duty to Save Lives	Empathy to Spare Dignity
Fearful of Death & Dying	Value-Conscious
Fight-or-Flight Reaction	Peaceful, Easy Feeling
Glass Half Empty	Glass Half Full
Deficits-Frustrations-Unfinished	Abundance-Satisfaction-Fullfillment
Oblige Others	Supported by Others
Medicare Entitlements	Palli-Care Enlightenment
Big Business	Personal Service
Buying Into the System	Bucking the System
Chance Living Longer	Prefer Dying at Home

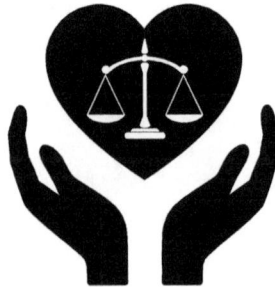

Check YES or NO to the following statements:

☐ **YES** ☐ **NO** **1.** You have an incurable illness, infection or cancer that involves a vital organ (brain, heart, lung, liver, stomach or kidney).

☐ **YES** ☐ **NO** **2.** You care more about feeling better than getting better.

☐ **YES** ☐ **NO** **3.** You can no longer live independently.

☐ **YES** ☐ **NO** **4.** Your family member has become your caregiver.

☐ **YES** ☐ **NO** **5.** You like to make your own choices.

☐ **YES** ☐ **NO** **6.** You don't invest time and energy in losing propositions.

☐ **YES** ☐ **NO** **7.** You are more comfortable at home than in the hospital.

☐ **YES** ☐ **NO** **8.** You don't like doctors or needles.

☐ **YES** ☐ **NO** **9.** You dread artificial life support and ICU admission.

☐ **YES** ☐ **NO** **10.** You prefer to be treated as a person rather than as a patient.

If you said YES to more than five statements, you will benefit from receiving palliative care.

Palliative care offers a kinder, gentler approach than the standard practice of medicine. Some people expect aggressive treatment of their illness, but those who receive palliative care believe "less is more." Less medical intervention and regulation affords more personal freedom and choice. People who enroll in this conservative approach begin to appreciate living fully while managing chronic illness.

Most people equate disease with treatment. Something bad happens (like a sore throat) and the doctor makes it better. When one of your major organs fails, the doctor can't make it better.

How do you guard against unnecessary treatment?

Are you required to suffer before your incurable disease takes your life?

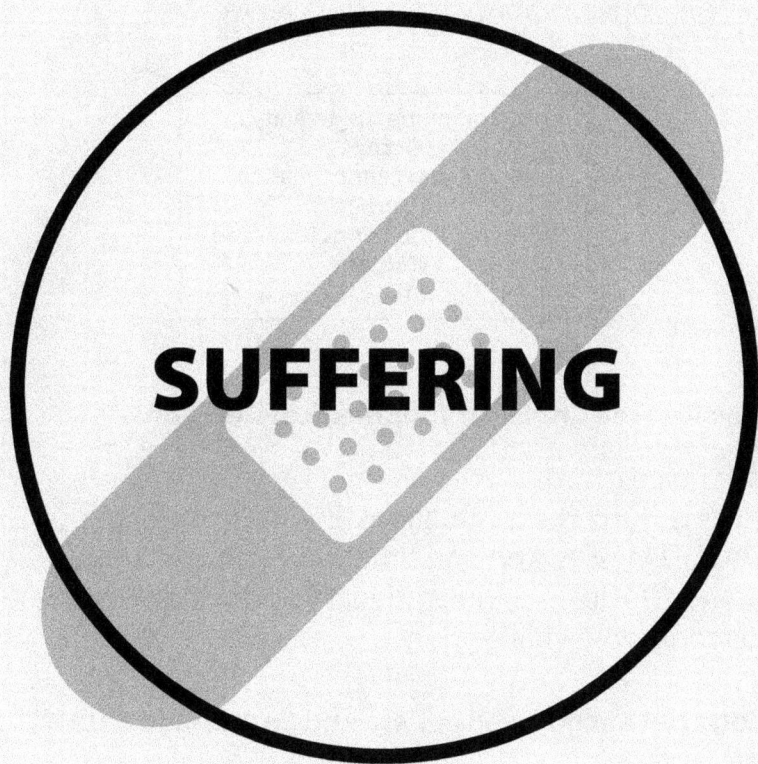

SUFFERING

Remove Suffering from the Disease Process

"Pain is inevitable, but suffering is optional"— even with end-stage disease. In fact, people live longer when they learn how to **cope with stress.** You have to know the difference between the things you cannot change (medical conditions) and the things you can (quality if life). This wisdom helps you accept an incurable illness and prompts conversations about stress reduction.

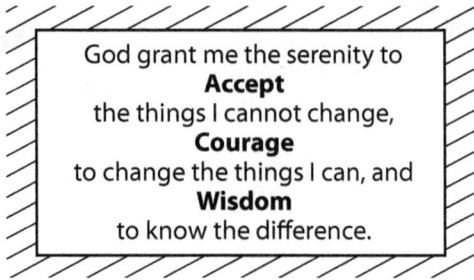

> God grant me the serenity to
> **Accept**
> the things I cannot change,
> **Courage**
> to change the things I can, and
> **Wisdom**
> to know the difference.

Allow for Free Choice in Your Medical Decisions

Free choice means there's no right or wrong answer, particularly in no-win situations. End-stage disease or terminal illness is a no-win situation. Feeling like you're "damned if you do and damned if you don't" makes these situations more challenging.

Bridge between Advance Care and End-of-Life Care

Medical complications often occur with incurable illness and the real possibility of death exists. **Decisions have to be made.** Do you continue to fight and risk falling into the troubling, raging waters of a horrific death - or use palliative care as the bridge to a peaceful death? It's often said, "We'll cross that bridge when we come to it." Since the possibility of death occurs with each emergency room visit, are you prepared to "crossover" the bridge? Do you have this option? Do you have home-based palliative care? If not, you'll be admitted to the hospital and chance a fate worse than death.

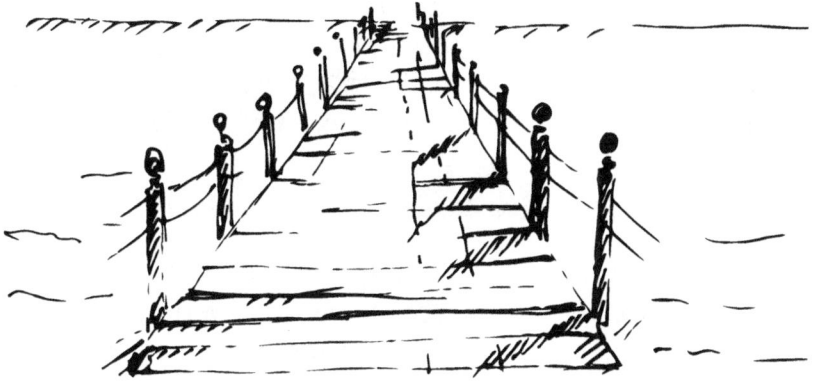

You will receive routine home visits and phone calls each month from your palliative nurse. These visits include a review of your medication and overall well-being. In addition, the **palliative nurse becomes your first responder,** 24/7. Your caregiver will have the nurse's contact information as an alternative number to 911, which will lessen the chance of your going to the emergency room and being hospitalized against your will.

A Higher Level of Care That Respects Your Wishes

Patients who receive advance care need to follow their doctor's orders. Those enrolled in palliative care inform the doctor of their wishes; they decide whether they receive better care in the hospital or at home. Hospitals have rules and regulations. You make the rules in your own home.

Feel Safe at Home

In baseball, home plate symbolizes the place we start and return to. You're generally considered safe at home and understand home is where the heart is. You often feel more comfortable in your own bed and make your best decisions after having time to "sleep on it." In addition, the patient who plays ball at home gains the home-field advantage.

Home-Based Palliative Care Allows You to be in Control

"Sometimes you feel like a nut, sometimes you don't." Based on what feels right, some days you want to be more active, and other days you want to rest. Your caregivers often take on the responsibility of keeping you alive, but they need to listen to you. When you are in control, the focus has to be on your wishes for the day.

What's the difference between being a "patient" and being a "person?" Often, "patient" means you're suffering. Something is wrong with you. Ideally, you would never be treated like this in your own home. As you try to do your best to manage the situation, you deserve respect over constant nagging.

Palliation Means Compassionate Treatment

What's the best thing you can do for a person nearing life's end? The answer is to show kindness and mercy. Some caregivers believe medical intervention is the answer to making patients better. The goal of palliative care is less medical intervention and more kindness. Talking to patients rather than testing for everything that could be wrong with them demonstrates compassion. This act of kindness cleanses your mind, body and spirit of feeling chronically ill.

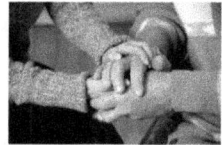

Live More Fully

For patients, the purpose of palliative care is to comfort your body, provide peace of mind and lift your spirit. Through your remaining days, you will hopefully think, "If I died at this moment, I would feel blessed." Appreciating what you can accomplish rather than what you cannot removes expectations. Hopes and dreams are replaced with love and gratitude.

Trust Yourself

Being *human* means you will die someday. Being *humane* means you can acknowledge your medical condition and can still love yourself. Faith, hope and love challenge you to never quit … to persevere. Strive to believe you're exactly where you should be in the circle of life. Remain open to the appropriate standard of care. Knowing where you stand in life allows you to maintain control of the situation and end life in peace.

Palliative Care Within the Circle of Life

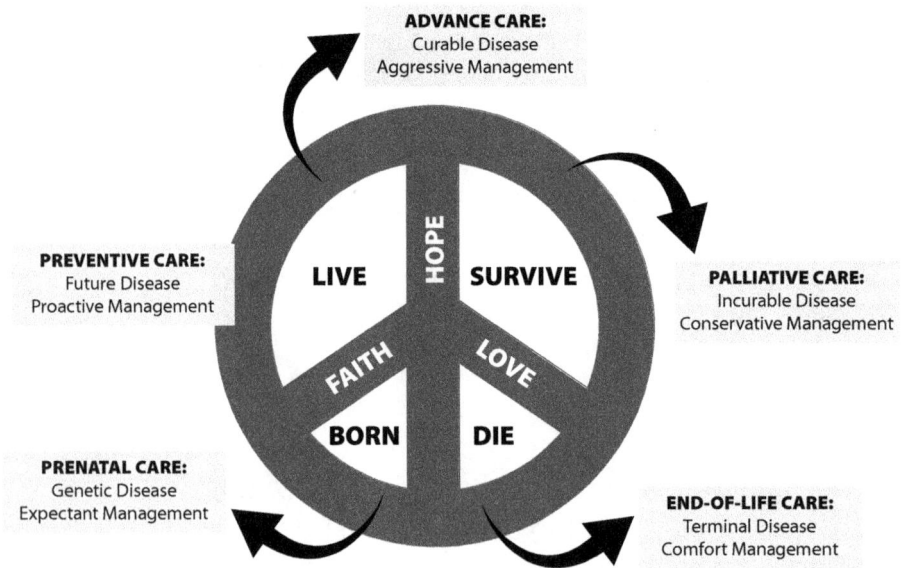

ADVANCE CARE:
Curable Disease
Aggressive Management

PREVENTIVE CARE:
Future Disease
Proactive Management

PALLIATIVE CARE:
Incurable Disease
Conservative Management

PRENATAL CARE:
Genetic Disease
Expectant Management

END-OF-LIFE CARE:
Terminal Disease
Comfort Management

LIVE HOPE SURVIVE
FAITH LOVE
BORN DIE

When there is No Cure for What Ails You

If you have a heart attack, you deserve all necessary treatment to prevent further damage. When you have heart failure along with a poor prognosis, CPR is ineffective. Palliative care offers peace of mind in your decision to not be resuscitated. When a door closes (with end-stage disease), another one opens (to receiving palliative care).

When You Receive Medicare

Medicare recipients are getting older and living longer. By the time you reach age 65, your doctor should have some idea of the health risks that will contribute to your death. This opens the discussion of what life expectancy means to you. Physicians who keep you in the dark are not your best advocates. If you don't express your final wishes upfront, you are guilty of keeping your physician in the dark as well.

When You Have a Caregiver

If you live independently, you deserve advance care. If you have a caregiver, provide them with a palliative care advocate (nurse). A palliative nurse is their best friend in supporting your interests.

When You're in Assisted Living

Assisted living means you will no longer die at home, but you could die in a hospital or nursing home. Palliative care allows assisted living to be the next best option to dying at home.

- Hospitals/Skilled-Nursing Facilities (prolonging your life)

- Assisted-Living Facilities (making living easier)

- Homecare Agencies (keeping you at home with family)

Palliative care educators often suggest a team approach for advanced illness management. You may want to guard against too many people telling you what to do. With home-based palliative care, you answer to only two people: **Your caregiver and the palliative care nurse.**

Your caregiver and the palliative nurse are the most valuable players on your team. Physicians rarely understand the concept of less being more. They tend to order tests to find every single thing that's medically wrong with you. A palliative nurse leaves well enough alone and focuses on your quality of life.

For most, this means keeping you at home and away from medical specialists and hospitals. Having two people representing your best interest is like having two parents. Sometimes they don't agree, but there is room for negotiation. No one wants to take full responsibility of another person's life-and-death situation. Having three people (including you) decide your fate lessens the burden and builds consensus.

How your medical condition is managed at home depends on two factors: the palliative nurse's resources and your caregiver's stamina. Ultimately, you need to consider the demands placed on your valuable players. You cannot expect advance care at home, along with skilled nursing. Home-based palliative care is only practical when you prefer to leave well enough alone. You're focused on easing any pain or shortness of breath without treating the underlying medical problem and prolonging life.

How is Palliative Care Different from Hospice?

Hospice is appropriate when you are in the final stage of dying. Palliative care supports your living at home while expecting to die. These two options are often given in tandem, but many insurance companies only provide hospice benefits. You might need to enroll in hospice to receive home-based palliative care. When life expectancy is fewer than six months, use hospice to your advantage by receiving more palliative care resources.

Hospice care reassures patients and their caregivers it's okay for them to rest in peace.

Many studies have shown people live longer while receiving palliative care. They often choose to spend more time with family and friends, take a trip or plan for their funeral. Those who choose to fight to the end often die sooner with less quality of life.

Palliative care allows you to live with vitality until you take a turn for the worse. Then, hospice care is appropriate, and you are essentially allowed to die in your sleep. **No heroics** are required in the transition between palliative care and hospice.

Palliative care gives patients permission to not be hospitalized.

Palliative care manages chronic illness, while hospice comforts the terminally ill. Only you can decide when a chronic illness becomes terminal, since physicians don't guess when you prefer to quit. You might use palliative care to begin the process of winding down your life. Weigh your quantity of years with your quality of life.

Quantity of Years
vs. Quality of Life

Quantity of years means prolonging life through more medication, procedures and misery—living as long as possible through continuing **medical treatment.**

Quality of life means choosing natural death by limiting medication, hospitalization and suffering—living with vitality by receiving **palliative care.**

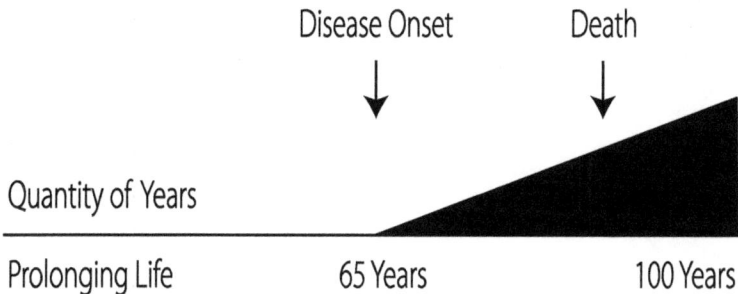

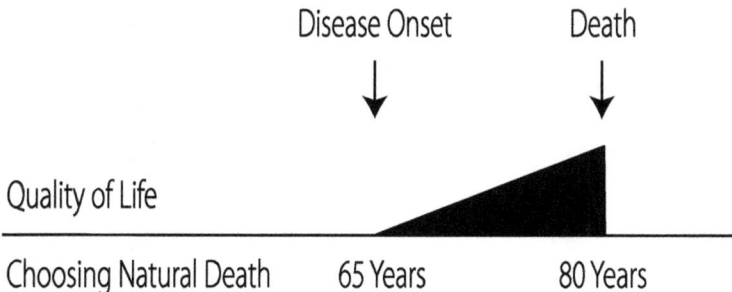

Disease Onset   Death

Quantity of Years

Prolonging Life   65 Years   100 Years

Disease Onset   Death

Quality of Life

Choosing Natural Death   65 Years   80 Years

19

This is a tricky question. It depends on the health coverage you have and whether the company understands the value of palliative care. Many companies provide home-based palliative care through hospice enrollment.

Some insurers are less concerned about paying for **person-centered care** and only cover treatments prescribed by your doctor. You're better served if your insurer allows you to have it your way: dying with dignity. Consider your palliative care concerns when selecting between:

■ Health insurance companies including Medicare and private payers.

■ Long-term health insurance.

Death can cause people — even physicians — to become alarmed, overreact and make bad decisions. This is how perfectly good people experience a fate worse than death and end up in intensive care units against their will. You don't want to be careless about dying — your final act — and palliative care allows you to have a say. It respects your final wishes.

Personal dignity suggests you value life and consider physical abuse demeaning. Dignity also helps you decide between self-preservation and self-validation, depending on your goals and personal values. Palliative care is less concerned about life and death. Its focus is on what's probably most important to you, allowing you to remain in control of your choices.

We all want to die

with dignity.

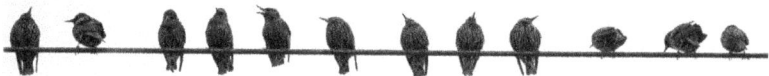

Palliative care provides the message, "Dignity is realized when you follow your heart and make your own choices." This self-respect is the certainty of being right in pursuing your final wishes.

Your self-determination and final wishes are key to taking control of your medical decisions.

Booklet Bonuses:

Your medical condition and physician might leave you with no choice but to stay in the hospital. Under the Patient Self Determination Act, you can always make the choice to safely return home.

Understand and claim your palliative care rights.

Your Palliative Care Rights

1. You have the right to sleep in your own bed tonight – without being disturbed or afraid of dying.

2. You have the right to let others manage your pain, nausea and difficulty breathing – with compassion.

3. You have the right to forget your past, present and future medical problems and resume living to the best of your ability.

4. You have the right to have others lift your spirit and allow you to be stress free.

5. You have the right to pursue your "beginning of the end" with humility, dignity and naturally.

**When you no longer have your health,
consider the next best option.**

Palliative Care 2.0
(Home-based palliative care)

**A 10-Point Plan That Outlines
Patient Goals and Personal Values**

1. Natural death beats artificial life support.

2. End-of-life conversations occur at the beginning of your chronic illness.

3. Advance planning prevents unwanted surgeries and ICU admissions.

4. Quality of life needs to be considered before unnecessary tests and procedures are ordered.

5. Your best interest overrules physicians' orders.

6. Home-based palliative care reduces your having to stay in the hospital.

7. Palliative care is considered a nursing practice, not a medical specialty.

8. Your patient/caregiver advocate (nurse) lessens the need for a medical team.

9. Spiritual well-being makes medical intervention unnecessary.

10. Personal dignity overcomes the fear of death and dying.

About Kevin Haselhorst, M.D.

Dr. Kevin Haselhorst enjoys a lively career as an emergency physician. While caring for those near the death, he has become painfully aware that our life journey rarely ends peacefully. Emergency room patients are typically burdened with multiple medical conditions, yet caregivers repeatedly have them admitted to the hospital in hopes of holding off the inevitable. The result: patients and caregivers becoming self-defeated and less in control.

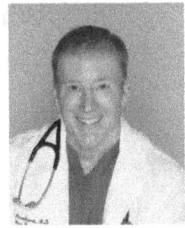

Dr. Haselhorst is the author of **Wishes to Die For,** which helps readers decide what's important to them as their health declines and how to specify the end-of-life care they expect from healthcare providers and family members. This book examines dying with dignity from medical and spiritual perspectives, discussing how to balance the hope of staying alive with the right to die humanely and peacefully.

Contact Dr. Kevin Haselhorst for Consulting or Speaking:
http://kevinhaselhorst.com/contact/

Connect with Dr. H on Facebook:
https://www.facebook.com/kevin.haselhorst.1

Free Tips to Help Caregivers

Subscribe to Dr. H's Clipboard
(Free, twice-monthly email tips on advance care planning):
http://kevinhaselhorst.com/signup/

If you're caring for a loved one with a serious illness, it's easy to let your wishes prevent your patient from dying with dignity. You must be careful about what you say and how you say it.

My pocket guide, **10 Phrases That Stop Patients from Dying with Dignity...and What to Say Instead,** is available at **KevinHaselhorst.com**.

Customize this booklet for your needs!

1. If you're a **caregiver,** give a copy to those you care for and those who care for you.

2. If you're a **palliative care company or organization,** give this booklet as an invitation to your services.

3. If you're an **insurance company**, promote the value of palliative care.

4. If you're a **primary doctor**, give your Medicare patients the gift of this booklet.

5. If you're a **medical specialist**, suggest that your patients have palliative resources.

6. If you're a **nurse**, you understand why patients need this booklet.

7. If you're a **social worker**, this booklet is like providing patients a best pal.

8. If you're a **hospital administrator**, allow this booklet to make patient care run smoothly.

9. If you're a **teaching institution**, this booklet needs to be required reading.

10. If you're a **spiritual community**, support those in need of palliative care.

Discount pricing for bulk orders | Licensing agreements available

Contact: DrH@KevinHaselhorst.com or
Call 480-907-6027